MALE AGING

BUSTED

Gregory A. Kevorkian B.S. M.A.

Dedication

This book is dedicated to my two sons, Drew and Jarad, with the hope that they may benefit from the research and information in this book to stay healthy and forestall the aging process and to my wife, Christine, who is always there to encourage me.

TABLE of CONTENTS

Introduction

Living in this century has given us the opportunity to benefit from the vast amount of research into anti-aging and the clinical use of anti-aging medicine.

The information in this book is not presented as a "how to" but as an informative reference for the very lay man approaching the critical age where all his bodily systems are going down the other side of the hill, as they say. For each topic addressed, it will be an overview, as there are whole books written for each one.

For the reader's protection a physician well versed in anti-aging methods should be consulted.

The reader needs to understand that when doing any anti-aging hormone therapy, levels are to stay within physiological ranges and not supra physiological levels (above the range). Levels should be brought to where they were at their peak, usually in the second decade of life, and a synergistic approach should be taken balancing HT (hormone therapy), diet, supplements and exercise.

I am sure there will be information that you "may" not understand. You should use that opportunity to research that area which will add to your knowledge. It is hoped that the information in this book will give you the desire to do what's necessary to slow down the aging process, avoid disease and live a healthier life!

Aging

Men reach a peak of growth and development in their mid 20s. After that peak, Mother Nature programs the body to begin aging until death. During aging there are quite a few changes that tax the body, disability is not necessarily a part of aging. Health and lifestyle factors, along with the genetics of the individual, determine the response to these changes. Many of the bodily functions that are affected by aging include:

- Hearing, which declines especially in relation to the highest pitched tones.
- The proportion of fat to muscle, which may increase by as much as 30%. Typically, the total padding of body fat accumulates around the stomach. The ability to excrete fats is impaired, and therefore the storage of fats increases, including cholesterol and fat-soluble nutrients.
- The amount of water in the body decreases, which therefore decreases the absorption of water-soluble nutrients. Also, there is less saliva and other lubricating fluids.
- The liver and the kidneys cannot function as efficiently, thus affecting the elimination of wastes.

- A decrease in the ease of digestion, with a decrease in stomach acid production.
- A loss of muscle strength and coordination, with an accompanying loss of mobility, agility, and flexibility.
- A decline in sexual functioning.
- A decrease in the sensations of taste and smell.
- Changes in the cardiovascular and respiratory systems, leading to decreased oxygen and nutrients throughout the body.
- Decreased functioning of the nervous system so that nerve impulses are not transmitted as efficiently, reflexes are not as sharp, and memory and learning are diminished.
- A decrease in bone strength and density.
- Thinning of the skin and wrinkling.
- Declining visual abilities.
- A compromised ability to produce vitamin D from sunlight.
- A reduction in protein formation leading to shrinkage in muscle mass and decreased bone formation, possibly leading to osteoporosis. [1]

Andropause is the time in many men's lives' when the hormones naturally decline. It is when there is a decline in a man's androgen levels usually occurring in their forties or early fifties. It has been said that it is analogues to Menopause in women.

As men approach middle age they begin to experience a gradual reduction in many of the above bodily functions. The most obvious are decreases in energy levels, memory, libido, hair, nails, skin, vision, hearing, insulin sensitivity, muscle mass and strength.

It is accepted by many that these changes are inevitable but researchers are finding that these changes can be slowed down and in some cases reversed to some degree. In their book, Stopping the Clock, Dr. Klatz and Dr. Goldman state, "The deterioration and vulnerability to the diseases of aging can be slowed, prevented and potentially reversed, memory loss, fatigue, heart disease, circulatory problems, arthritis, Alzheimer's disease and cancer." Diabetes can also be included.

Researchers are now finding ways to intervene in the breaking down of our bodily systems and interrupt the aging/disease cycle. We no longer have to accept this decline in physical and mental functioning!

Some Important Areas of Research

Tissue Regeneration and Organ Cloning:

This area of biotechnology is focusing on how to repair damaged tissues and exploring the possibility of cloning new organs from our own DNA.

Organs grown from our own tissue would be easily accepted by the body. This would eliminate the need for the patient to take organ rejection medication for the rest of their lives. Advanced tissue regeneration technology may enable us to repair and revitalize any tissue or organ system within the body.[2]

Human Adult Stem Cells:

Stem cells are often called pluripotent cells meaning that they can change into any cell type in the body. The advantage of stem cell research is exploring the potential of these cells to create revolutionary therapies and treatments.[2]

Telomeres and Aging:

Telomeres are part of the connecting tissue within each living cell. These strands get shorter with each cell division. Leonard Hayflick studied this phenomenon. The Hayflick Limit now refers to the concept that each cell has a certain limited number of cell divisions before the cell dies. Telomerase is an enzyme that protects the length of the telomere. Could more telomerase in our cells help us live longer?

Current telomerase research is being conducted to see if cell division capability can be maintained resulting in a longer human lifespan. Telomere research may also help in tissue engineering since it helps regulate cell division.[2]

Longevity Lifestyle Strategies

This is a broad area of anti-aging research that includes life extension supplements, anti-aging drugs, and anti-aging therapies, i.e. hormone replacement therapy (HRT). Simple lifestyle changes, must focus on getting optimal levels of nutrition, plenty of regular exercise, and deep relaxation.[2]

Some of the Longevity Lifestyle Strategies of research will be the focus of this book.

A Very Short Cholesterol Primer

Cholesterol, from the Ancient Greek *chole-* (bile) and *stereos* (solid) followed by the chemical suffix *-ol* for an alcohol, is an organic molecule. It is a sterol (or modified steroid), and an essential structural component of animal cell membranes that is required to establish proper membrane permeability and fluidity.[3]

In addition to its importance within cells, cholesterol also serves as a precursor for the biosynthesis of steroid hormones, bile acids, and vitamin D. Cholesterol is the principal sterol synthesized by animals; in vertebrates it is formed predominantly in the liver.[4]

Within cells, cholesterol is the precursor molecule in several biochemical pathways. In the liver, cholesterol is converted to bile, which is then stored in the gallbladder. Bile contains bile salts, which solubilize fats in the digestive tract and aid in the intestinal absorption of fat molecules as well as the fat-soluble vitamins, A, D, E, and K.

Cholesterol is an important precursor molecule for the synthesis of vitamin D and the steroid hormones, including the adrenal gland hormones cortisol and aldosterone, as well as the sex hormones progesterone, estrogen, testosterone, and their derivatives.[4]

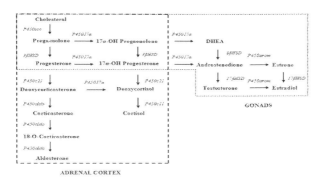

ADRENAL CORTEX

Cholesterol is essential for all animal life; however normal and particularly high levels of fats (including cholesterol) in the blood circulation, *depending on how they are transported within lipoproteins*, are strongly associated with the progression of atherosclerosis, which is a thickening and hardening of arteries.

For a man of about 150 pounds, typical total body-cholesterol synthesis is approximately 1,000 mg per day, and total body content is approximately 35 g, primarily located within all the cells of the body. In the United States, typical daily intake of additional cholesterol is 200–300 mg.[5]

Most ingested cholesterol is poorly absorbed. The body also compensates for any absorption of additional cholesterol by reducing cholesterol synthesis.[6]

It isn't in the scope of this book to go into all aspects of lipid metabolism, discussing HDL, LDL, etc. etc, but it is very important to understand the many roles cholesterol plays in the functioning of the body, **especially the formation of hormones.**

It's a lot About Hormones

A hormone (from Greek ὁρμή, "impetus") is a chemical released by a cell, a gland, or an organ in one part of the body that affects cells in other parts of the organism. Only a small amount of hormone is required to alter cell metabolism. In essence, it is a chemical messenger that transports a signal from one cell to another.

Hormones are secreted by a collection of glands inside the body known as the "endocrine system." (A "gland" is a group of cells that produces and secretes chemicals into the body.) The major glands that make up the endocrine system include the hypothalamus, the pituitary gland, the thyroid and parathyroid, the adrenals, the pineal body, and the ovaries and testes (the "gonads").

"As the body ages, the pituitary's ability to produce stimulating hormones slows down. Likewise, the glands that respond to stimulating hormones slow down. The result is an overall decline in hormone levels."[7] In a great percentage of older men there is a reduction in Thyroid hormones, DHEA, (Dehydroepiandrosterone), Testosterone, Growth Hormone, Melatonin and an increase in Estrogen. Estrogen overload is a serious problem in aging men. "One report showed that estrogen levels of the average 54-year-old man are higher than those of the average 59-year-old woman."[8]

Over fifty different hormones have been identified in the bodies of humans, and more are still being discovered. Hormones influence and regulate practically every cell, tissue, organ, and function of our bodies, including growth, development, metabolism, maintenance/balance of our internal environment (homeostasis), and sexual and reproductive function.

As we go forward, we will address some of the main hormones in men that researchers feel can be adjusted to slow down the aging process. In his book the "Miracle of Natural Hormones" Dr. David Brownstein states, "Although there is no cure for aging, my clinical experience has shown that natural hormones, when used appropriately, can slow down many of the signs of aging including deteriorating mental function, loss of muscle tone, and wrinkled skin."

As men reach mid life many experience the same process as women do during Menopause; they begin to experience a decline in many of their hormone levels. Men reach their peak in hormone production in their twenties and the level of hormones drop steadily as they age.

The main hormones that we will be discussing which are relevant to male aging are Thyroid hormone, DHEA (Dehydroepiandrosterone), Testosterone, Growth Hormone and Melatonin. All these hormones are available either by prescription or over the counter and can be used to adjust hormone levels to thwart the aging process. It is felt by many anti-aging practitioners that hormone levels should be brought back to their peak levels, usually during the second decade of life.

Thyroid

Thyroid gland: A gland that makes and stores hormones that help regulate the heart rate, blood pressure, body temperature, and the rate at which food is converted into energy. Thyroid hormones are essential for the function of every cell in the body. They help regulate growth and the rate of chemical reactions (metabolism) in the body. Thyroid hormones also help children grow and develop.

The thyroid gland is located in the lower part of the neck, below the Adam's apple, wrapped around the trachea (windpipe). It has the shape of a butterfly: two wings (lobes) attached to one another by a middle part.

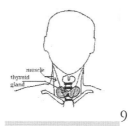

The thyroid uses iodine, a mineral found in some foods and in iodized salt, to make its hormones. The two most important thyroid hormones are thyroxine (T4) and triiodothyronine (T3). Thyroid stimulating hormone (TSH), which is produced by the pituitary gland, acts to stimulate hormone production by the thyroid gland. The thyroid gland also makes the hormone calcitonin, which is involved in calcium metabolism and stimulating bone cells to add calcium to bone.[10]

According to the AACE (American Association of Clinical Endocrinologists), the number of people affected by Thyroid Disease now surpasses the number of people diagnosed with Diabetes or Heart Disease.

- 27 Million: The number of Americans estimated to suffer from Thyroid Disease.
- 13 Million: The number of Americans estimated to suffer from Thyroid Disease…but remain undiagnosed.[11]

As you read these statistics, it is safe to say that you may know someone that has Thyroid disease, Hypothyroid, (low thyroid) or Hyperthyroid, (overactive Thyroid). Hypothyroid will be the focus since we are addressing anti-aging and decline in hormones. The below chart traces the decline of Thyroid hormone as we age.

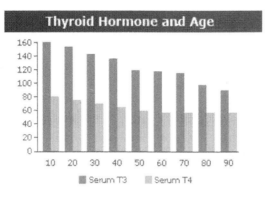

Thyroid Hormone and Age

Serum T3   Serum T4

12

Hypothyroidism is a condition characterized by abnormally low thyroid hormone production. As stated above, the two most important thyroid hormones are thyroxine (T4) and triiodothyronine (T3). However, the hormone with the most biological activity is T3. Once released from the thyroid gland into the blood, a large amount of T4 is converted into T3 - the active hormone that affects the metabolism of cells.

The thyroid itself is regulated by another gland that is located in the brain, called the pituitary. The pituitary is regulated in part by the thyroid (via a "feedback" effect of thyroid hormone on the pituitary gland) and by another gland called the hypothalamus. The hypothalamus releases a hormone called thyrotropin releasing hormone (TRH), which sends a signal to the pituitary to release thyroid stimulating hormone (TSH). In turn, TSH sends a signal to the thyroid to release thyroid hormones. A deficiency of thyroid hormone (hypothyroidism) can be caused by a disruption at any one of these levels.

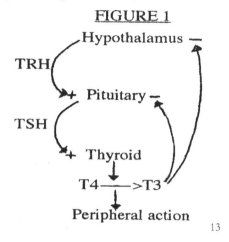

FIGURE 1

The rate of thyroid hormone production is controlled by the pituitary gland with the release of TSH. If there is an insufficient amount of thyroid hormone the release of TSH is increased by the pituitary gland to stimulate more thyroid hormone production.

If there is an excessive amount of circulating thyroid hormone, TSH levels are reduced, as the pituitary attempts to decrease the production of thyroid hormone. In persons with type 1 hypothyroidism, there is a persistent low level of circulating thyroid hormones.[14]

The reader should understand that Thyroid hormone can affect basically every system in the body.

Some Major Symptoms of Hypothyroidism:

- Fatigue

- Weakness

- Weight gain or increased difficulty losing weight

- Coarse, Dry hair

- Dry, rough pale skin

- Hair loss

- Cold intolerance (you can't tolerate cold temperatures like those around you)

- Muscle cramps and frequent muscle aches

- Constipation

- Depression

- Irritability

- Memory loss

- Abnormal menstrual cycles

- Decreased libido

A person need not exhibit all the symptoms to have Hypothyroidism and may have only some, such as fatigue or cold intolerance.

Diagnosing Hypothyroid Disease:

The main tests used by physicians to diagnose Hypothyroidism are TSH, (thyroid stimulating hormone), T4, total and free, T3, total and free.

The reader needs to be made aware that despite the sensitivity of all the tests the doctors can give a patient today, a mildly hypothyroid person can still appear normal in these tests.

Many people have symptoms of hypothyroidism and are clearly hypothyroid, yet they complain that no doctors will help them. Even if their tests come up "normal", they suffer tremendously with symptoms of hypothyroidism daily.

Why is it that so many people who need some thyroid help simply cannot get it from their doctor?

Dr. Richard Shames author of the book, "Thyroid Power" believes; "one reason so many people cannot get thyroid therapy is because many physicians are not aware of the excessive prevalence of low thyroid in the population, or of its collective toll on the nation's health".

The Mayo Clinic has determined that as much as 10 percent of the population suffers from thyroid problems and it appears to be on the increase. TSH tests and blood tests are useful to help diagnose hypothyroidism but should not be used alone. *Symptoms are the most important factor.*

It is rare that a blood chemistry panel shows your true condition because the values measured are only about 30% accurate. It is common for a hypothyroid person to have a completely normal thyroid panel. This is why the Thyroid Panel is considered by many to be inadequate. It is also common for a hypothyroid person to have a low TSH value, which is usually interpreted as hyperthyroidism, not the reverse, despite many symptoms of low thyroid (depression, dry skin, weight problems, chronic infections, hair loss, low blood sugar, and so on). TSH tests are not as scientifically accurate as they need to be! [15]

Treating Hypothyroidism: Main Stream Physicians

After taking the appropriate test, TSH, T4, T3 etc, and determining that the patient has hypothyroidism, the main stream physician will usually treat the condition with the synthetic thyroid hormone, levothyroxine (for example, Synthroid, Levoxyl, or Levothroid). Testing is usually done every 4 to 6 weeks until the physician feels that the patient's blood levels are in the acceptable range.

It can't be stressed enough that blood test are not the end all of treatment. How the patient feels is the deciding factor.

Many doctors refuse to look outside the box and accept that a patient may need more thyroid hormone than a test range calls for.

As Mary J. Shomon, a patient advocate and thyroid patient herself, said in the Times article, *"What's normal for me may not be normal for you. We're patients, not lab values."*

An alternative approach: Why the difference?

In his book"Hypothyroidism, Type 2: The Epidemic" Dr. Mark Starr has an interesting hypothesis and treats his thyroid patients accordingly. He explains that there are two types of hypothyroidism, Type 1 and Type 2.

> With Type 1 Hypothyroidism, the thyroid does not produce sufficient amounts of hormone to maintain "normal" blood levels of hormones, which in turn will maintain normal blood levels of thyroid-stimulating hormone (TSH) produced by the pituitary.

> With Type 2 Hypothyroidism, the thyroid gland produces

"normal" amounts of hormone, but the cells are unable to utilize the hormone properly. Some experts call this thyroid hormone resistance (which may be regarded as similar to insulin resistance). Laboratory tests showing inadequate bloodstream levels of thyroid hormone make it easy to diagnose, Type 1 hypothyroidism. However, lab tests fail to detect Type 2 hypothyroidism, because despite adequate bloodstream hormone levels, the cells are unable to accept and utilize that hormone. Since the main problem lies with the cells that are actually utilizing the hormone, a different approach needs to be taken when testing for – and to a certain extent, when treating – Type 2, hypothyroidism.

Dr. Mark Starr writes that in the early twentieth century:

> …the ultimate test of whether or not a patient was hypothyroid was the patient's response to a trial of thyroid hormones. Confirmation depended upon improvement or resolution of their symptoms. . . . [But] the list of thyroid blood tests grew until there were scores of available tests. Unfortunately, they failed to improve the ability to detect Type 2 hypothyroidism.

> Dr. Starr goes on to say, "The most common blood test for hypothyroidism depends on the following assumptions. The body tissues transmit their need for

thyroid hormones to the hypothalamus in the brain, which sends a signal to the pituitary gland. In turn, the pituitary secretes thyroid stimulating hormone (TSH), which signals the thyroid gland to secrete more hormones. These hormones are then carried by the bloodstream to the tissues. The action of the thyroid hormones on the tissues reduces the tissue signals to the brain for more thyroid hormones, and the pituitary stops secreting TSH. The problem with this scenario is that most of the time, the mitochondria in toxic and defective cells are unable to convey to the brain their need for thyroid hormone, even if it's urgently required. In fact, according to numerous studies, people whose mitochondria tested abnormal nonetheless had normal thyroid hormone levels in their blood. Modern thyroid blood tests, Starr reminds us, do not detect Type 2 hypothyroidism because thyroid hormone levels [in the bloodstream] may be normal, but they are not high enough to stimulate the defective mitochondria into normal activity. Nor are the blood thyroid hormone levels high enough to induce the resistant receptor sites on the cells to start accepting hormone. Any part of the cell can be involved in the failure to process and utilize thyroid hormone.

There is no scientific evidence, Starr bluntly states, after providing a detailed review of the literature, to support the doctor's claim that the TSH test detects hypothyroidism in the vast majority of patients."[16]

Treating Hypothyroidism: The alternative!

Dr. Broda Barnes, one of the pioneers in thyroid therapy, Dr. Mark Starr and a host of alternative physicians take a different approach to treating hypothyroidism.

Dessicated Thyroid

In the1960s, people suffering from hypothyroidism were given desiccated thyroid derived from pigs. This means the entire dried gland and its contents – all four forms of thyroid hormone, RNA, DNA, and other co-factors. But by the 1970s, isolated thyroxin (T4) was introduced as the "gold standard" of thyroid medications.

By definition, thyroxin is only a portion of the thyroid hormone complex. Since it does not contain the synergistic effects of the entire glandular material, not surprisingly, it proved less effective clinically than the desiccated thyroid.[17]

Treatment begins with small doses of desiccated thyroid with testing usually every 4 to 6 weeks. Blood tests, clinical observation of symptoms, along with basal temperature testing is evaluated, if symptoms persist and basal temperature remains low, under 98.2° an increase of ½ grain (30 mgs) is administered every 4 to 6 weeks, until symptoms are alleviated or basal temp exceeds the prescribed limit. Some alternative physicians may also use creams containing T4 and T3 and the testing procedure is the same.

There is one simple thing almost anyone can do at home to uncover a possible underactive thyroid:

Take your own basal temperature.

The "basal body temperature" test was developed by Broda O. Barnes, M.D.

Because thyroid hormone is so vital to cellular metabolism, reduced thyroid function often manifests as a drop in body temperature to below the normal level of 98.6*F. Barnes recommended the following procedure: "Immediately upon awakening, and with as little movement as possible, place the thermometer under the tongue or in the rectum. Leave it there for 10 minutes. Record the readings on three consecutive days. If the average temperature over the three days is less than 97.8*F, then, you may have hypothyroidism. Even if you have had a blood test and were told you did not have a low thyroid reading, you might go back and look at the test results again. You may find that your blood levels of thyroid hormones are actually at the lower end of the normal range. Many people who are within the so-called "normal" range but below the midpoint "may" benefit enormously from thyroid supplementation."[18]

Whatever method a patient chooses to follow, it is wise to keep in mind **that reaching a state of normalcy and the alleviation of symptoms is the goal and not numbers on a blood test!**

Finding a physician who is willing to listen and work with the patient and not limit themselves to blood levels is an important part of addressing Hypothyroidism!

All the prescribed treatments for Hypothyroidism, synthetic thyroid, desiccated thyroid and creams are by prescription from a physician.

Dhea: Dehydroepiandrosterone

Dehydroepiandrosterone is an important endogenous steroid hormone. **It is the most abundant circulating steroid in humans,** in whom it is produced in the adrenal glands, the gonads, skin and the brain, where it functions predominantly as a metabolic intermediate in the biosynthesis of the androgens, **Testosterone** and **Estrogen**. However, DHEA also has a variety of potential biological effects in its own right, binding to an array of nuclear and cell surface receptors, and acting as a neurosteroid.[19]

DHEA (*dehydroepiandrosterone*) is produced by your adrenal glands. Dr. William Regelson, the most noted of DHEA researchers, calls it the "mother hormone" because "it is the precursor (foundation or raw material) needed for the production of other hormones, including our major sex hormones." Unfortunately, DHEA levels peak in the body at the age of 20 and then rapidly decrease. At age 40, most people secrete only 33% of what they produced when they were young. In our 60's and 70's, we have only 5 to 10% of our original level. The graph of this decline closely matches the increase of the killer illnesses of cancer and heart disease.

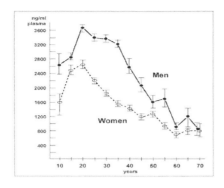

The above graph shows the decline in Dhea as we age.

Dr. William Regelson also states that "DHEA is a bio-marker for aging and it declines in a linear fashion with the progression of aging. If you're going to approach aging rationally, you have to bio-quantitate human aging. DHEA, as a bio-marker for aging, is one of the best indicators of how old you really are."

He goes on to say "I have spent more than twenty five years researching DHEA and prescribing it to patients. It restores energy, improves mood, increases sex drive, enhances memory, relieves stress, reduces body fat, and even makes your skin softer and your hair shiner. I think that just about every adult age forty-five or older can benefit from taking DHEA"

Dhea and Dhea Sulfate:

Both DHEA and DHEA-S are steroid hormones that the body uses as a starting point in the production of other hormones in both men and women.

The body can alter DHEA to make DHEA-S. DHEA-S is made naturally from DHEA in the liver by the addition of a sulfate molecule. The body produces much more DHEA-S compared to DHEA each day: While the body makes only about 1 to 2 mg of DHEA, it produces between 10 and 15 mg of DHEA-S.

DHEA-S is much more stable in the body than DHEA. This is because the kidneys remove DHEA and DHEA-S from the blood but clear DHEA-S at a much slower rate than DHEA, leaving more DHEA-S remaining in the body. If your doctor suspects that you may have a deficiency in DHEA or DHEA-S, the level of DHEA-S will likely be tested due to its stability.[20]

In the book "The DHEA Breakthrough" by Stephen Cherniske the author lays out the following chart in regard to **DHEA-S** levels.

Men

Prime Peak: 450-600

Good: 300-450

Deficient: 125-300

Worrisome: Less than 125

After getting your DHEA-S blood levels taken, using the above chart, you can see what category you fall into.

It was noted above that DHEA affects many functions in the body. Below several specific areas will be addressed that affect older men.

Cardiovascular Disease:

There is a clear relationship between DHEA levels and cardiovascular disease.

As DHEA declines, the incidence of cardiovascular disease rises in men (Barrett-Connor 1987; Herrington 1990; Hautanen 1994; Barrett-Connor 1995; Feldman 1998) and in women (Johannes 1999).

Diabetic men with the lowest DHEA levels have a significantly greater chance of developing coronary heart disease (Fukui 2005). The risk of death is higher among those with the lowest levels of DHEA in men less than age 70 (Mazat 2001). DHEA plays a protective role in the development of atherosclerosis and coronary artery disease (Gordon 1988; Eich 1993), especially among men. Several mechanisms are involved: inhibition of G6PD (which can modify the lipid spectrum), suppression of platelet aggregation, and reduced cell proliferation (Porsova-

Dutoit 2000). Men with lower DHEA-S are more likely to have atherosclerosis (Herrington 1990) and calcified deposits in the abdominal aorta (Hak 2002). Because cortisol increases the risk of heart attack and the severity of atherosclerosis in men (Laughlin 2000), raising DHEA levels to increase the DHEA/cortisol ratio has promise for reducing cardiovascular risk (Barrett-Connor 1995). Low DHEA is related to premature heart attack in men (Mitchell 1994). Severely ill cardiac patients and those with acute heart attack have lower DHEA levels for as long as 3 to 4 months after the event (Slowinska-Srzednicka 1989; Ruiz 1992).[23]

Cognitive decline:

One of the most distressing elements of aging is the loss of mental "sharpness." Once again, DHEA has been shown to improve measures of cognitive function in laboratory studies (Roberts 1987; Flood 1988). Abnormal balances in the brain between DHEA-S and cortisol have been shown to decrease brain function (Kalmijn 1998; Ferrari 2001).[23]

Diabetes:

DHEA appears to increase insulin sensitivity. Insulin resistance is an early indicator of type 2 diabetes and is closely associated with obesity, which are both major risk factors for heart disease.

A decrease in DHEA-S is associated with the development of type 2 diabetes (Kameda 2005). [23]

Metabolic Syndrome:

Metabolic Syndrome is characterized by several conditions, which are all associated with elevated risk for heart disease (e.g., increased insulin resistance, obesity, and abnormal cholesterol levels). In metabolic syndrome, these individual risk factors act synergistically, raising the risk of heart disease higher than their individual risk levels alone. Although research is still continuing, scientists have linked elevated cholesterol to lower DHEA levels (Nestler 1992). Long-term DHEA supplementation improves insulin sensitivity by 30%, raises high-density lipoprotein (HDL) cholesterol by 12%, and lowers low-density lipoprotein (LDL) cholesterol by 11% and triglycerides by 20% (Lasco 2001). The lowering of LDL by DHEA has an antioxidant effect, which could have anti-atherogenic consequences (Nestler 1988; Nestler 1991; Kurzman 1990; Khalil 2000). DHEA also decreases abdominal fat, an important characteristic of metabolic syndrome (Villareal 2000; Villareal 2004).[23]

Stress:

DHEA protects your body from the hormone cortisol and the stress that triggers its production. Like DHEA, cortisol is secreted by the adrenal glands. If over secreted, cortisol injures your body's tissues. When you're under stress, your adrenal glands release large amounts of cortisol. People under chronic stress have high cortisol levels (unless their adrenal glands have already burned out, in which case their cortisol levels are low). The presence of too much cortisol leads to age-accelerating damage. As stress accumulates over decades, cortisol levels tend to rise as well. Many people over age 40 have elevated cortisol.

DHEA and cortisol have an inverse, or adversarial, relationship. When you're faced with prolonged stress, your cortisol/DHEA ratio--a measure of health status and aging--can rise by a factor of 5. This means that the excess cortisol is battering DHEA's protective shield. DHEA supplementation increases your stress tolerance, lowers your cortisol/DHEA ratio, and protects you against cortisol-induced cellular damage.[24]

Immune system:

A recent study found a strong inverse correlation between human serum DHEA-S levels and interleukin 6 (IL-6) levels. IL-6 is one of many cytokines, or immune cell "quasi-hormones," which collectively regulate immune activity. High interleukin levels are implicated as a causal factor in many diseases, such as rheumatoid arthritis, osteoporosis, B-cell cancers, atherosclerosis and Parkinson's disease. Interleukin 6 levels tend to dramatically increase with aging, just as DHEA-S levels decrease with aging. After studying 120 healthy human subjects, 15-75 years of age, R.H. Straub and colleagues concluded: "decreased DHEA serum concentrations during aging or inflammatory diseases will be paralleled by a significant increase in interleukin production. Thus, we conclude that the decrease in DHEA levels is a deleterious process, in particular during chronic inflammatory diseases." O.Khorram, L.Vu and S.S.C. Yen, long-time DHEA researchers, published an important DHEA study in 1997.

Nine healthy "age-advanced men" (mean age: 63) were given DHEA daily for 20 weeks after 2 weeks' placebo treatment. They noted that the study demonstrates the stimulatory effects of DHEA on the immune function of age-advanced men. DHEA rejuvenated the immune system by increasing the secretion of IL-2, a potent T-cell growth factor, increasing the number of cells expressing the IL-2 receptor, and enhancing T cell responsiveness to mitogen stimulation, all of which decline during physiologic aging. The significant increase in NK [natural killer] cell cytotoxicity in DHEA treated subjects was potentially related to the increased number of NK cells, both events being mediated by DHEA-induced IL-2 stimulation. There were no adverse effects noted with DHEA administration.[25]

Skin:

Most DHEA metabolism actually occurs in the largest organ of the body, the dermis, the skin. Many metabolic processes go on in the skin – consider where vitamin D is made and processed by the body - the skin. DHEA is much the same.

Research studies show that higher levels of DHEA not only make people healthier, and happier and more productive. People have more energy, get more done and are in a better mood.

Medical research supporting these benefits of DHEA are widely known, but what is not commonly known is the medical research studies that also show DHEA is also very good for the skin.[26]

A study performed by Dr. Calvo, Dr. Labrie, et al at the CHUL Research Center at Laval University found that DHEA increased production of sebum, better known as "skin oil". Sebum not only contributes to smooth supple skin; it also contains a number of antimicrobial features that protect the skin from infections and irritations[26]

Dr. Lee, Dr. Oh, and Dr. Kim at Keimyung University School of Medicine showed that DHEA switches on multiple collagen producing genes and at the same time reduced genes associated with hardening or toughening of skin that forms calluses and rough skin.

The researchers concluded that DHEA could have an anti-aging effect on the skin from stimulation of collagen production and improved structural organization of skin cells.[26] Further medical research done by Dr. Brandner, Dr. Kief and their team at the University Hospital in Hamburg Germany have demonstrated how DHEA also improves skin "brightness" and counteracts the thin 'papery' appearance of aging skin, that is a noticeable visible sign of aging. Furthermore, DHEA helps reduce risks of both ultraviolet and chemically induced skin cancer.[26]

Who should not take Dhea?

- People under the age of 35 (unless following the advice of their physician). In general young people are already producing adequate DHEA. Since the hormone can be converted to testosterone and estrogen, taking DHEA can produce symptoms associated with excess sex hormones, such as acne.
- Pregnant or nursing women.
- Men with prostate cancer.

7- Keto Dhea:

Because 7-Keto is not converted into estrogen or testosterone, it may be the perfect complement to DHEA therapy, as well as providing an option for people who have hormone dependent cancers!

Among DHEA's many metabolites, one has attracted significant attention for its unique ability to lower cholesterol, burn fat, and improve the immune system. This metabolite is known as 7-Keto DHEA.

Scientific studies have shown that 7-Keto can help people burn fat through a process known as "thermogenesis."

This means the body's metabolic rate is accelerated, generating heat and energy that consumes calories and burns fat. 7-Keto accomplishes this by boosting the levels of liver enzymes that stimulate fatty acid oxidation.

In one study of 30 overweight adults, study subjects received 100mg of 7-Keto twice daily or placebo. They also participated in a supervised exercise and diet program. At the end of the study, those taking 7-Keto lost 6.3 pounds on average, versus 2.1 pounds for the control group (Kalman 2000).

7-Keto has also been studied for its immune-boosting and cholesterol-lowering properties. In a study on cholesterol levels, human volunteers applied a gel containing 25mg of 7-Keto for five consecutive days. At the end of the study, the subjects taking 7-Keto experienced a rise in good HDL cholesterol and a slight reduction in harmful LDL cholesterol (Sulcova 2001).

Another study looking at immune function found that four weeks of 7-Keto supplementation improved immune function in elderly men and women. In this study, subjects over age 65 took 100mg of 7-Keto twice daily or placebo. The subjects on 7-Keto experienced a significant decrease in immune suppressor cells and an increase in immune helper cells (Zenk 2004).[27]

Dhea and 7-Keto Dhea are over the counter supplements.

Testosterone

You hear it all the time on TV and radio, are you tired, no energy, lost your desire for sex, have erectile dysfunction, bad mood, depression and have increased fat around your middle. You may have low T!

Testosterone is produced in the Leydig cells of the testicles and most of it is secreted into the bloodstream, travelling to locations as distant as the brain. Some testosterone remains in the testicles themselves, helping to produce an environment conducive to the production of mature sperm.

Testosterone is an anabolic steroid. Anabolic steroids are chemicals that cause anabolism, an overall increase in protein production and storage, primarily seen as an increase in muscle and bone. The opposite of anabolism is catabolism, which is seen during starvation, for example, when the body starts breaking down protein in muscle to provide nutrients for the rest of the body.[28]

When people hear anabolic steroids they immediately think of athletes, especially bodybuilders, who many times use dosages which put them far above the normal limits.

The Statistics on Low Testosterone:

The number of men with low testosterone levels is expected to go up as the number of older American men increases. Here are some statistics:

- Fifteen to 30 million American men have erectile dysfunction.
- As many as 13 million American men may have low testosterone.
- Seventy percent of men with low testosterone report erectile dysfunction and 63 percent say they have a low sex drive.
- About one-third of men with diabetes may have low testosterone.
- Ninety percent of men with low testosterone receive no treatment.[29]

As testosterone levels decline, many men feel as though they're "getting old" much faster. In fact, many symptoms, once considered a natural part of the aging process like lethargy, depression, irritability, sexual dysfunction, and mood swings, may actually be the low testosterone symptoms. Sound familiar? In men, the low testosterone levels lead to andropause often referred to as "Male Menopause".

300 nanograms/dl is the standard testosterone limit below which it is termed as low testosterone, and at this level or higher, you may experience the symptoms of low T. As we mentioned before, you should get your levels up to what they were in your 20ies. Testosterone decline and low testosterone symptoms are common with the aging process. Starting around the age of 35 to 40, testosterone levels (Total T) in men, decline by roughly 1% each year." [30]

The Chart depicts the declining levels of Testosterone

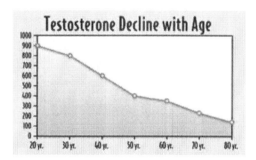

Low testosterone levels involve many low testosterone symptoms that deteriorate the life of a suffering man.

Some symptoms of declining testosterone are,

- Visible belly fat
- Trouble in orgasm
- Testicular shrinkage

- Loss of energy and stamina
- Less fuel for a man's sex drive
- Feeling of depletion at day end
- Irritability with family and friends
- Loss of muscle mass from arms and legs
- Low production of fluid containing sperms
- Gloomy feeling with lowest optimism level
- Lack of "electricity" (Numbness) in the genital area
- Erectile dysfunction (impossible erections or failure in ejaculation)

Low testosterone levels occur due to many reasons; major low testosterone causes are following:

- Obesity
- Testicle injury
- Infectious diseases
- Excess of blood iron
- Inflammatory diseases
- Natural process of aging
- Chemo/radiation treatment
- Performance boosting Drugs
- Pain or hormonal medication

Take the "Is it Low T?" Quiz

1. Do you have a decrease in libido (sex Drive)?

Yes ⊙ No ⊙

2. Do you have a lack of energy?

Yes ⊙ No ⊙

3. Do you have a decrease in strength?

Yes ⊙ No ⊙

4. Have you lost height?

Yes ⊙ No ⊙

5. Is there a decrease in your enjoyment of life?

Yes ⊙ No ⊙

6. Are you sad and/or grumpy?

Yes ⊙ No ⊙

7. Are your erections less strong?

Yes ⊙ No ⊙

8. A deterioration in your ability to play sports?

Yes ⊙ No ⊙

9. Are you falling asleep after dinner?

Yes ⊙ No ⊙

10. Is there deterioration in your work?

Yes ⊙ No ⦿ 52

Testing for low T:

If you are experiencing the symptoms of low testosterone, your physician can determine whether you actually have low T and a possible cause, by some simple blood tests.

Total Testosterone

Free Testosterone

SHBG (Sex Hormone Binding Globulin)/ Albumin

Estrogen / Estradiol

LH (Lutenizing hormone)/FSH (follicle-stimulating hormone)

PSA

CBC

The following is a description of the relevance of the above tests.

Total testosterone:

Measures the amount of total testosterone in the blood. Total T in itself is not a true measure of a man's testosterone status.

Free Testosterone:

Makes up about 1 to 2 % of the total testosterone and is a good indicator of what is available to the cells.

SHBG and Albumin:

Serves as a transport carrier, shuttling testosterone to sex hormone receptors *throughout* your body. It thus acts as the master regulator of your sex hormone levels, maintaining the delicate balance between estrogen and testosterone is critical to overall health in aging humans.

As you age, SHBG levels may steadily **rise**, even though your production of sex hormones (testosterone) continues to **decline**. The result, SHBG binds to what few sex hormones you have remaining and reduces their bioavailability to the cells in your body.

With elevated SHBG in the blood, too much testosterone may be sequestered and thus functionally unavailable to healthy tissues. Because testing for SHBG is largely overlooked, many older men (and their doctors) may be led to believe through "standard testing" that they have "normal" total testosterone levels—but since most of it may be bound to elevated levels of SHBG, in actuality they may be **Testosterone Deficient!**

Why? Testosterone, like all steroid hormones, is derived from cholesterol, a fat molecule. Fats don't dissolve in water, so the amount of free testosterone floating in your bloodstream is small (about 1-2% of the total amount). Most of the circulating testosterone in your blood is either bound to the protein albumin or to SHBG.

As a result of imprecise testosterone measurement, aging men may experience signs of feminization as their increased SHBG binds testosterone, preventing testosterone from exerting its effects and leaving estrogens' physiological impact on the male physiology unchecked. [31]

Estrogen / Estradiol:

Aromatase is an enzyme found in the liver, responsible for the conversion of the androgens androstenedione and testosterone into the estrogens, estrone and estradiol. Lowering the production of aromatase can cause the body to produce less estradiol and maintain a higher testosterone state. The main side effect in men from too much estrogen is gynecomastia. Gynecomastia is enlargement of the glandular tissue of the male breast. Anti-Aromatase supplements and medications are used to suppress aromatase and prevent more estradiol from being produced.

Other factors known to increase aromatase activity include age, being overweight, insulin production, insulin levels, and alcohol consumption.

Aromatase inhibitors are being prescribed to men on testosterone replacement therapy (TRT) as a way to keep estradiol levels from increasing when testosterone is introduced. Increasing your testosterone may results in an increase in estradiol; **this in turn will shut off some of the testosterone effects.**

Aromatase is primarily concentrated in the skin, especially over fat, in the scrotum, and around the nipples. Excess fat cells can contribute to an increased amount of aromatase, and nutrient deficiencies can also produce higher levels. Lowering the production of aromatase will preserve and stimulate more free testosterone.

Some common causes of increased aromatase activity:

- Aging
- Zinc deficiency
- Obesity
- Carbohydrate intolerance and insulin sensitivity
- Overuse of alcohol
- Liver function changes
- Prescription Drug side effects, especially diuretics and liver activity drugs

LH (Lutenizing hormone)/FSH (follicle-stimulating hormone):

These are referred to collectively as the gonadotrophins. They can help the doctor determine what may be causing low testosterone.

PSA:

This test is used primarily to screen for prostate cancer. A PSA test measures the amount of prostate-specific antigen (PSA) in your blood. PSA is a protein produced in the prostate, a small gland that sits below a man's bladder. PSA is mostly found in semen, which also is produced in the prostate. Small amounts of PSA ordinarily circulate in the blood.

John Crisler D.O. states "While the possibility of inducing, or increasing, the symptoms of BPH (Benign Prostatic Hypertrophy) is often mentioned, numerous studies have shown this is not the case. TRT has also been shown to not increase the risk of prostate cancer as well.

On the subject of prostate cancer, that is one of two medical conditions which are, at this time, an absolute contraindication (meaning a reason to withhold treatment) to TRT. That is why doctors who administer TRT monitor prostate health with regular PSA tests and Digital Rectal Exams. The other contraindication is male breast cancer."

"There's a recent opinion developing that prostate cancer has more to do with estrogen than with dihydrotestosterone, which is actually created from testosterone combining with a common enzyme in your body. This theory is that many men, as they age, convert too much testosterone to estrogen and

that this excessive estrogen is the cause of prostate enlargement or prostate cancer.''32

If this opinion is valid then taking anti-aromatase medication or supplements which lower estrogen should help to prevent prostate cancer.

CBC:

This test is taken to monitor the level of red blood cells. Testosterone helps to stimulate the production of red blood cells. An overabundance of red blood cells, Erythrocytosis, can make the blood too thick which may lead to stroke or heart attack!

Treating Low T: There are several common methods to treat low T.

Injections:

One of the most common types of treatments is testosterone injections, which is injected into a muscle usually once or twice weekly.

You can give yourself these injections or have them done by a physician. Injections are a very effective way of replacing your testosterone, but do come with side effects you should be aware of. This form of replacement therapy shuts down the natural production of testosterone in your body and you will need to go through a "post therapy" in order to kick start your own production again.

This will usually be done through HCG injections or something similar. This type of treatment can also lead to highs and lows in your body's testosterone as it will peak shortly after each injection and slowly decline until the next one since your body is producing little to no testosterone on its own.

Testosterone Pellets:

The next option would be testosterone pellets, which are placed under the skin around the hip area and testosterone is released gradually into the body.

These pellets dissolve evenly without the highs and lows of the injections. Unfortunately, an incision has to be made in your skin in which to place the pellets, this is usually done every three to six months. Some of the documented side effects have been an extrusion rate of 8% - 12% depending on the study, bleeding and infection.

Testosterone Creams and Gels:

There are also testosterone creams and gels that you can apply topically. These creams and gels can be effective, painless and no incisions are necessary. The main drawback to using creams or gels is that you can accidentally transfer the testosterone to other people via skin to skin contact.

Determining which method would be a decision between you and your doctor. Effectiveness, convenience and cost are some of the determining factors. Some health insurance companies cover testosterone replacement.[33]

Some supplements to boost Testosterone:

Herbs for Testosterone

The use of herbs has been a proven safe, effective way to enhance health through the centuries. These herbs for testosterone can be used on their own or in conjunction with other herbs and natural remedies, and sometimes they can be used as an enhancement to medical treatments or prescription medications.

1. Sarsaparilla Root

This is a natural steroid that helps increase muscle mass in both men and women. It also helps with prostate problems and offers sexual enhancement for men. It can also help with male pattern baldness. This herb can be taken in capsule form and can be increased over time if it doesn't seem to be effective enough with the first level dose. As an added bonus, you can supplement the capsule with drinks that contain the herb.

2. Tongkat Ali

Also known as Long Jack, this herb from Malaysia and Indonesia has been proven to help enhance sexual performance for men. It has also been proven to increase muscle mass, boost energy levels, improve concentration and memory, and provide more endurance and stamina. This can be taken in conjunction with other herbs for testosterone.

3. Yohimbe Bark

Originating in Africa, this herb can boost energy levels and is especially great for athletes who need more stamina. It can be helpful for those who are on medications for depression, as it helps counteract the sexual problems that are often associated with anti-depressant use. In addition to the enhanced testosterone levels, it is also believed to increase oxygen to the body, thus easing heart problems.

4. Maca Root

This plant from the Andes increases testosterone and other hormones that are essential to reproductive health. As a result, libido rises and energy levels go up. This herb is also great for improving muscle mass. This can be used in conjunction with other herbs for testosterone, and it can also be found in some drinks. This was considered such a potent remedy that it was reserved only for Inca royalty for many centuries.

5. Ginseng

One of the most common herbs for testosterone and other problems, ginseng has been proven to improve energy levels, enhance memory and boost sexual function for both men and women. The Chinese believe that ginseng can also improve longevity. This can be found in many supplements sold over the counter.

6. Tribulus Terrestris

Also known as Puncture Vine, this herb is from India and parts of Eastern Europe. It has been seen to work in a matter of days by raising testosterone levels, improving sports performance, and serving as an aphrodisiac. It apparently works very well, as chimps that were given this herb saw testosterone increases of over 50 percent.

7. Mucuna Pruriens

This herb is both a growth hormone and a natural steroid, thus enhancing testosterone levels. This herb increases the dopamine in the brain, thus encouraging the body to create more testosterone on its own. It also decreases prolactin levels, which have been shown to be a key player in sexual dysfunction in men.

8. Horny Goat Weed

Just as the name suggests, this herb has been used to increase libido and improve sexual stamina for over 2,000 years. Not only does it increase testosterone levels, it also helps open up the blood vessels, which can lead to more energy and increased vitality.

9. Muira Puama

From the Brazilian rainforest, this herb has been used for centuries by natural medicine doctors and shamans in South America. It enhances testosterone production in men, thus leading to increased energy, lower chances of depression, better mental acuity and increased libido. It has also been shown to be an aphrodisiac.

10. Fo Ti

This Chinese herb has been used for thousands of years as a way to turn back aging, promotes longevity and enhances sexual health. Also known as Hoshou Wu, it has also been a cure for impotence for many centuries.

Please keep in mind that you should consult a doctor before taking any of these treatments. Problems with low testosterone can be caused by some medical conditions, so treating the underlying causes can remedy the problem. The only way to know for sure is to consult your physician before beginning any sort of natural treatment.[34]

Some estradiol lowering supplements to boost free testosterone:

Zinc: Zinc can slow the change of testosterone into estrogen so taking a zinc supplement can help lower the level of estrogen in a man's body. Other antioxidants will also help slow the conversion of testosterone.

Indole-3-Carbinol or I3C is found in cruciferous vegetables. It helps detoxify estrogens because it works very well with estrogen blockers.

Diindolylmethane or DIM is a metabolite of I3C. It is stronger and more effective compound which increases the amount of good estrogens, while reducing the amount of bad estrogens and xenoestrogens. When you take DIM, you may notice a change in your urine color. Those are the toxins and estrogens being flushed out from the body. The best time to take it is before bed or after you wake up since hormone levels are raising at night, during sleep.

Chrysin (5'7-DihyDroxyisoflavone) is a flavonoid from blue passion flower which has shown to be the most powerful natural aromatase inhibitor. However, its low bioavailability gives weak results in real life. To overcome that, you should consume it with piperine from black pepper, dihydroxybergamottin (DHB) from grapefruit or both.

Nettle Root contains probably the weakest of all Aromatase inhibitors, 3,4-Divanillyltetrahydrofuran and Secoisolariciresinol. Nettle root does help free up testosterone by binding to the SHBG[35]

Exercise and Testosterone:

6 Ways to Increase Testosterone with Exercise

Tip #1: Sprint

Multiple studies have shown that you can boost your testosterone levels by sprinting. In one study, testosterone levels increased significantly for people who performed a series of very short (but intense) 6-second sprints – and testosterone levels remained high even after those people had fully recovered from the sprint workout.

So how can you implement the strategy of sprinting to increase testosterone? Try performing several sprints on the treadmill after you've lifted weights at the gym, or just head out into the backyard, a park, or your neighborhood block and do a few sprint repeats on your days off from weight training. You can even do your sprints on a bicycle or elliptical trainer. Try to include 5-10 short sprints when you do a sprint workout, sprint no longer than 15 seconds, get full recovery after each sprint (generally 3-4 times longer than you actually sprinted), and do a sprint workout 2-3 times a week for optimal results.

Tip #2: Lift Heavy Stuff

While you can do high reps with low weights or low reps with high weights, studies have shown that it definitely takes heavy weights to significantly boost testosterone. Full body, heavy exercises like **squats**, **dead lifts**, **bench presses**, and **Olympic lifts** should ideally be used, at 85-95% of your 1RM (or one repetition maximum). You need to do 2-3 full body weight lifting workouts per week to get good testosterone-boosting results.

If you're a beginner or new to weight training, don't let this concept of heavy lifting scare you away. You can simulate many of these exercises on weight training machines until you're strong and skilled enough to perform the free weight barbell or dumbbell versions.

Tip #3: Use Long Rest Periods

Scientists have studied the effects of very short rest periods on testosterone and found that longer rest periods of around 120 seconds between sets are better for building testosterone (although you can still build other hormones, such as growth hormone, with shorter rest periods).

Considering what you've just learned about lifting heavy weights, this makes sense, since the shorter your recovery periods, the less weight you're going to be able to lift. However, it can seem like a waste of time to be sitting on your butt for 3 minutes between each exercise.

So if your goals are to increase testosterone, it is recommended that you maximize your time at the gym by doing alternate activities during these long rest periods, such as stretching, or better yet, exercises that don't stress the same muscles you just worked.

For example, you can do one heavy set of bench presses, recover for just 30-60 seconds, and then do one heavy set of squats. Go back and forth until all your sets are done, and you'll get twice as much done in half the time, while still getting the testosterone boosting benefits of lifting heavy and long rest periods.

Tip #4: Do Forced Reps

To do a forced repetition, you perform a weight lifting exercise for as many reps as you can, and then have partner (a "spotter") assist you with completing several additional repetitions (anywhere from 1-5 extra reps).

Research shows that this type of forced rep set generates more testosterone than simply doing as many reps as you can do by yourself.

It's best to do forced reps with a multi-joint, large motor movement exercise. For example, you can do a warm-up set of barbell squats, then, with a partner, a personal trainer, or someone you ask at the gym to help you, choose a weight that allows you to do 5-6 repetitions on your own, but requires an assistant to get another 3-4 reps done after that, for a total of 8-10 reps. You can repeat this for anywhere from 2-6 sets.

While you don't need to perform forced reps for every workout or set that you do, if you're trying to increase testosterone, it can be especially helpful to do your last set of any exercise as a forced rep set.

Tip #5: Use Your Legs

In another study that investigated the hormonal response to weight training, participants were split into an arm-only training group and a leg-plus-arm training group. Testosterone increases were significantly higher in the group that added lower body training to their upper body training.

While it can be tempting, especially for guys, to focus on exercises like biceps curls and bench pressing, you'll notice far better results for lean muscle mass, energy, sex drive, and fat loss when you include multi-joint leg exercises such as lunges and squats into your regimen.

So here's an example of a full body workout you could do 3 days per week to boost testosterone:

Warm-up

- 4 sets of 8 repetitions **bench press**, paired with 4 sets of 8 repetitions **squats**.
- 4 sets of 8 repetitions **dead lifts** paired with 4 sets of 8 repetitions pull-ups.
- 6 sets of maximum 10 second **sprints**.
- Cool-down

Tip #6: Avoid Chronic Cardio

Long endurance sports such as cycling seem to lower testosterone in the same way that weight lifting and weight training seem to increase it. For example, one 2003 study found that testosterone levels were significantly lower in cyclists than age-matched weightlifters, or even an untrained control group. Some researchers have even concluded that this type of low testosterone in endurance athletes is an adaptation that gives cyclists or runners a competitive advantage – since the extra muscle mass from testosterone would probably slow you down.[36]

Human Growth Hormone

Recently in the news we hear about athletes and movie stars who are using Human Growth Hormone to look younger and maximize their performance. What is HGH and what does it do?

Growth hormone (**GH** or **HGH**), also known as somatotropin or somatropin, is a peptide hormone that stimulates growth, cell reproduction and regeneration in humans and other animals. Growth Hormone is specific only to certain kinds of cells and it is a 191-amino acid, single-chain polypeptide that is synthesized, stored, and secreted by somatotropic cells within the lateral wings of the anterior pituitary gland.[37]

David Brownstein M.D. states " The beneficial effects of using physiological doses of human growth hormone include improving and perhaps reversing many of the following signs of aging: thinning hair, wrinkled skin, loss of muscle tone, low resistance to stress, depression, low resistance to infection, poor healing of wounds, and varicose veins. Human growth hormone has also been shown to improve the following conditions: cardiac disease, fatigue, osteoporosis and perhaps cancer."

As with most hormone, HGH declines with age as illustrated in the following graph.

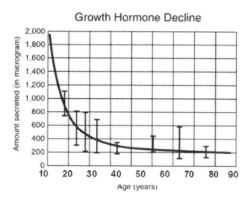

Growth Hormone Decline

Along with this decline come all the accompanying problems.

As stated above, growth hormone is made in the pituitary gland, which is located at the base of the brain.

It does a lot more than just make a child grow taller; it's responsible for the growth of the body, including organs and bones, and it helps the body's metabolic processes.

When growth hormone is released from the pituitary gland, it "tells" the liver to release a second hormone, called insulin-like growth factor-1 (IGF-1).

Together, growth hormone and IGF-1 tell the bones, muscles, and other organs and tissues to grow by adding more cells.

Detecting low growth hormone is by blood test for the levels of IGF-1.

The History of Human Growth Hormone:

The history of HGH has its origins in the 1920's. Once human growth hormone deficiency was discovered in humans, researchers have quickly tried to come up with a form of treatment. The first step in the lengthy history of HGH was rBGH or bovine growth hormone.

Scientists turned to cows for help and began extracting what growth hormone they could. They purified BGH as best they could and gave it to patients with Type-1 diabetes and hormone deficiencies.

Bovine growth hormone has a different molecular structure than the human hormone. This made most attempts at treatment unsuccessful. When BGH failed to work, one researcher turned to human cadavers for answers.

The History of HGH and Cadavers:

Situated in Boston, Massachusetts is Tufts University. An endocrinologist employed by the school named Maurice Raben, put the task of finding a successful treatment for HGH deficiency upon himself.

Raben turned to cadavers for help and began extracting human growth hormone from the pituitary gland of an autopsied body. He was successful in his venture in many ways.

First, he was able to extract enough HGH for treatment. Then he successfully purified enough of the hormone to administer to his first patient suffering from human growth hormone deficiency.

His first patient was a young man only 17 years old. The year was 1958 and Raben, along with his medical breakthrough, made history of his own. He successfully treated the boy. Some argue this is when the history of HGH was really made.

Human Growth Hormone Extraction from Cadavers Catches On:

When the 1960's rolled around, many endocrinologists had heard, read and studied about Maurice Raben and his successful treatment of human growth hormone deficiency and wanted to secure their own place in the history of HGH.

A large number of endocrinologists from around the country began contacting their local morgues and securing the pituitary glands of cadavers. The human growth hormone they were extracting came to be called cadaver-GH.

A National Pituitary Agency is Born:

The National Pituitary Agency has its place in the history of HGH. In 1960 the agency was formed by the U.S. National Institutes of Health.

The agency's purpose was to control the procurement and distribution of HGH.

Soon, other countries followed suit and established their own agencies to keep procurement and distribution safe, fair and legal. In the U.S., the National Pituitary Agency took control over a large scale effort to procure and distribute human growth hormone.

Only endocrinologists on a selective list received the HGH. During this part of the history of HGH, cadaver-GH was mainly used to treat hormone deficiencies in children. Typically, only children with severe cases of the deficiency were treated.

Once the child reached a certain height, treatment stopped. There was only so much cadaver-GH to go around. At this time many people as well as pharmaceutical companies were under the impression that the government controlled the procurement, distribution and allowed usage of cadaver-GH.

During the 1970's era of the history of HGH, a pharmaceutical company from Sweden began selling the first commercial human growth hormone product. The company, named Kabi, called their product Crescormon and began advertising to the public.

Cadaver-GH Hits a Standstill:

In 1985 the popularity surrounding cadaver-GH came to a halt. Four patients that were treated with cadaver-GH in the 60's had been diagnosed with Creutzfeldt-Jakob Disease, better known as CJD.

By 2003 the number of patients who had been treated with cadaver-GH and who now had CJD had risen to twenty-six. This has lead to the discovery of other CJD patients who had also received some form of GH treatment in their youth.

Cadaver-GH has not been used in humans since.

Synthetic Human Growth Hormone Hits the Market:

It wasn't until 1981 that a synthetic version of the human growth hormone hit the market. Genentech, an American pharmaceutical company, in collaboration with Kabi, developed a synthetic version of the hormone.

They called it rhGH, which stands for recombinant human growth hormone. The two companies used human growth hormone synthesis, referred to as Inclusion Body Technology, to create their product.

Today, thanks to much research and many advances, the process is called Protein Secretion Technology, also referred to as Somatropin. This remains the most commonly used form of HGH synthesis.[38]

Does HGH Treatment Work?

In July 1990, Dr. Daniel Rudman published his landmark clinical findings on the effects of HGH in the *New England Journal of Medicine*. The results were exciting and startling!

Effects of HGH in Men Over 60 Years of Age:

The declining activity of the growth hormone-insulin-like growth factor 1 (IGF-1) with advancing age may contribute to the decrease in lean body mass and the increase in mass of adipose tissue that occur with aging.

Trial Methods Used by Rudman:

To test this hypothesis, Dr. Rudman, studied IGF-1 plasma while working with volunteers aged 61 to 81 at the Medical College of Wisconsin-Milwaukee. Dr. Rudman used HGH manufactured synthetically to replicate what is created naturally in the body's own pituitary gland.

During the treatment period, 12 men (group 1) received approximately 0.03 mg of biosynthetic human growth hormone per kilogram of body weight subcutaneously, under the skin, three times a week, and 9 men (group 2) received no treatment.

Plasma IGF-1 levels were measured monthly. At the end of each period, Dr. Rudman's team measured lean body mass, the mass of adipose tissue, skin thickness (epidermis plus dermis), and bone density at nine skeletal sites.

Observations

Of the group who received treatment, their mean plasma IGF-1 levels rose back to youthful ranges **(500-1500 U/liter),** while the second group remained below **(350 U/liter).**

Also, in the group that received treatment for six months, it was observed that they showed an 8.8 percent increase in lean body mass, a 14.4 percent decrease in adipose-tissue mass, and a 1.6 percent increase in average lumbar vertebral bone density. Skin thickness increased .1 percent. The second group showed no significant change in lean body mass, the mass of adipose tissue, skin thickness, or bone density during treatment.

Dr. Rudman's Conclusions:

Diminished secretion of growth hormone is responsible in part for the decrease of lean body mass, the expansion of adipose-tissue mass, and the thinning of the skin that occurs in old age. (New England Journal of Medicine, 1990; 323:1-6)

In middle and late adulthood, all people experience a series of progressive alterations in body composition. The lean body mass shrinks and the mass of adipose tissue expand. The contraction in lean body mass reflects atrophic processes in skeletal muscle, liver, kidney, spleen, skin, and bone.

These structural changes have been considered unavoidable results of aging. It has recently been proposed, however, that reduced availability of growth hormone in late adulthood may contribute to such changes.

These alterations in body composition caused by growth hormone deficiency can be reversed by replacement doses of the hormone, as experiments in children, and adults 20 to 50 years old have shown. These findings suggest that the atrophy of the lean body mass and its component organs and the enlargement of the mass of adipose tissue that are characteristic of the elderly result at least in part from diminished secretion of growth hormone. If so, the age-related changes in body composition should be correctable in part by the administration of human growth hormone, now readily available as a biosynthetic product.

Since Dr. Rudman's initial findings, thousands of additional studies have supported the fact the HGH not only retards aging, but reverses the process as well.[39]

Cost of HGH treatment:

HGH treatment can cost anywhere from $800 to $2,500 a month, and usually require one or two self administered injections a day. The expensive cost of HGH prescription injections has primarily limited their use to the rich and famous.

Homeopathic HGH: A Low Cost Alternative?

Homeopathy, or homeopathic medicine, is a medical philosophy and practice based on the idea that the body has the ability to heal itself. Homeopathy was founded in the late 1700s in Germany and has been widely practiced throughout Europe. Homeopathic medicine views symptoms of illness as normal responses of the body as it attempts to regain health.

Homeopathy is based on the idea that "like cures like." That is, if a substance causes a symptom in a healthy person, giving the person a very small amount of the same substance may cure the illness. In theory, a homeopathic dose enhances the body's normal healing and self-regulatory processes.

A homeopathic health practitioner (homeopath) uses pills or liquid mixtures (solutions) containing only a little of an active ingredient (usually a plant or mineral) for treatment of disease. These are known as highly diluted or "potentiated" substances. There is some evidence to show that homeopathic medicines may have helpful effects.[40]

In the book, "Feeling Younger with Homeopathic HGH" by Dr. Howard Davis there is a quote from the father of HGH, Dr. Howard Turney. It reads as follows: "my wife and I have been using (homeopathic HGH) ... for some time now ... and we are receiving the benefits we were previously experiencing with the injectable form of HGH and at a greatly reduced price." You would never have a quote from a reputable doctor such as Dr. Howard Turney, who is the father and an expert in human growth hormone studies, concerning such important benefits using homeopathic human growth hormone, if homeopathic human growth hormone did not succeed or worked poorly.[41]

One of the key features of homeopathic medicine is to take a very insignificant amount of an herb or some other substance and put it into the body of someone that is suffering a disease or condition that has incredibly alike properties to the herb or molecule. The line of reasoning goes that since homeopathic HGH does not even use this principle in homeopathic medicine, it hence has all the more reason to be understood as something that does not succeed. Homeopathic human growth hormone, on the other hand, does use a number of the most important features of homeopathic medicine. The key homeopathic feature used with homeopathic human growth hormone involves a complex process of repeated vibrations of the liquid in which the very little quantity of the human growth hormone molecule is suspended. It is supposed that a trivial amount of HGH molecule suspended in this fluid has its properties transferred to the smaller molecules of the liquid through this complex process of repeated high vibrations to the liquid. The problem is that this is all theory and seems to go against the known values of science that such an insignificant quantity of HGH could possibly increase IGF-1.

The other drawback with the HGH molecule when used as a liquid spray for under the tongue is that it is too large of a molecule to infiltrate under the tongue. However, because the properties of the human growth hormone molecule are supposed to be infused to other smaller molecules there is then the capacity for these smaller molecules to diffuse under the tongue into the bloodstream with the matching abilities that are that of the HGH molecule. The skeptics argue that this is all theory and has no backing or proof in science. However, their argument is also not scientific, to conclude that on the grounds that we do not scientifically understand the process, it might not be factual. The fact is that there are many processes that cannot be scientifically understood or observed in their out workings and yet are scientifically observed with benefits that are proven real. Take for instance, the HGH molecule which numerous scientists concluded might not work because; they assumed it was scientifically impossible to infiltrate the blood brain barrier due to the fact that it was too large a molecule. Nonetheless, when they administered human growth hormone injections and did a tap on the backbone for fluid coming from the brain they discovered an abundance of human growth hormone molecules. This obviously revealed that the human growth hormone molecule in some mysterious way was able to diffuse the blood brain barrier.[42]

What to Look for in Homeopathic HGH Spray:

Homeopathy works on the basis of the electromagnetics and vibrations of the active ingredient, making it a much deeper form of medicine than modern allopathic medicine. For this reason you should not try to apply or compare allopathic measurements such as nanograms (ng), milligrams (mg), etc., to homeopathic products. Proper homeopathic products are only measured in potencies, not in nanograms, milligrams, etc.

In homeopathic measurements you will see a number in front of the letters X or C. This is the potency (strength) of the ingredient. The letter **"X"** indicates a 1 to 10 dilution and the letter **"C"** indicates a 1 to 100 dilution. The number in front of the letter is the number of times the ingredient has been diluted and succussed, which is what, potentiates the ingredient. As a general rule, the potency of an ingredient increases with each succussion and dilution. The key to effective homeopathic medicine is finding the potency that the body responds to best.

When looking for a human growth hormone product read product information and labels carefully and understand what they mean. Some products give the number of nanograms (ng) of HGH on the label. A nanogram is 1 billionth of a gram. Such a product is not a real homeopathic. Homeopathic products are not measured in nanograms, grams or other similar measurements and you should not find this on the label of a truly homeopathic product.

FDA registered homeopathic products will only give the proper potency (X and C) of the ingredient on the label, which is what makes the product effective.

Claimed Effects of HGH Spray:

According to Dr. Howard A. Davis different people notice different benefits. Some see immediate, dramatic results while others experience more subtle benefits. With proper diet and exercise he says the results can be faster, deeper and more pronounced. He states that many people have begun a whole new life on homeopathic HGH therapy.

General Expected Benefits in the 1st Month Include:

- Improved stamina
- Vivid Dreams
- Improved sleep, and feeling more refreshed upon awakening
- More optimistic attitude
- Increased energy (some report they feel 16 again)
- Better sense of humor

General Expected Benefits in the 3rd Month Include:

- Same as month one but heightened, some manifestations are exceptional
- Mental processes improve, desire to complete projects
- Muscle size increases, if the individual exercises
- Hair growth
- Increase in sexual desire
- Greater body flexibility
- Less pain

General Expected Benefits in the 5th Month Include:

- Impressive weight loss and reduction of inches, since fat is reduced and muscle tissue is increased and toned
- Improvement in skin texture and appearance (including skin discoloration)
- Thickening of skin and greater elasticity
- Reduction of the appearance of wrinkles
- Thickening of hair with a shiny and healthy appearance

Please note, around the fifth month, at times the body may shift into neutral and some results seem to diminish or vanish. Your body may be using HGH to rebuild tissue or, to a degree, be resting. Tests indicate that, after a while, you should see a resumption of the benefits and even some vast improvements.

General Expected Benefits in the 6th Month Include:

- Same as previous months, but better, with more consistent results. This is the exciting stage!
- Cellulite greatly diminishes
- Body is much more contoured
- Eyesight greatly improved

- Better emotional stability
- Stronger resistance to colds, flu and other illnesses
- Some pain and soreness disappear
- Old wounds have healed or are healing
- Excellent exercise tolerance
- Grayed hair begins to return to natural color
- Medical tests show a reduction in cholesterol (LDL) and triglycerides
- Blood pressure normalizes
- Heart rate improves
- Some conditions due to disease vanish or are diminished
- Immune system improves
- With proper diet and exercise, the results may be faster, deeper and more pronounced!

He also states that everyone is different, so you should consider the condition you were in before taking the product and how long you have been in that condition.

Lastly, he says that whether you notice immediate results or not, according to experience the homeopathic HGH should still be working. [43]

Growth Hormone Boosting Supplements:

GABA: An amino acid that stands for Gamma-Aminobutryic Acid, GABA is a very unique amino acid in that it actually acts as a neurotransmitter, rather than aiding in protein synthesis, like many other amino acids. When people say "amino acid" they are normally referring to alpha amino acids however GABA is not an alpha amino.

Some pre-workout supplements are beginning to include GABA in the mix. Of course you can also buy GABA in the powdered or pill form which is a good option because you can take larger doses that way. Of all of the natural growth hormone boosters, GABA is probably the most highly regarded.

Amino Acids: Other amino acids that have a "growth hormone boosting" effect include Ornithine, Lysine, Glutamine BCAA's, Taurine and Arginine. Taking these amino acids together in sufficient amounts can produce noticeable results.

There are supplements that include all of these amino acids along with other HGH and testosterone boosting ingredients. Amino acids are the basis for all supplements that aim to naturally increase HGH levels.[44]

Growth Hormone Boosting Exercises:

Resistance Training

Resistance training provides the highest exercise-induced growth hormone response (EIGR). How high the response is depends on the load and frequency of the training. When a person lifts heavier loads with the least amount of rest time possible, he causes the greatest amount of HGH to be released. Resistance exercises that require the largest muscle groups to be utilized, like lunges and squats, cause the greatest HGH release, because there are more muscle fibers being utilized, resulting in a greater anaerobic response.

Sprinting

HGH has a pulsatile release, making shorter bouts of exercise the best for HGH release. Pulsatile release means that it does not release on a constant or steady basis; instead, it releases in pulses. Therefore, sprinting (running, biking, swimming, among other exercises) for 10 minutes several times a day is very beneficial for HGH release. This allows the body to reach the highest lactic acid threshold possible and makes the muscles use the HGH the best.

Endurance Training

Endurance training will cause the release of HGH to vary according to intensity, duration and frequency. It will also depend on the type of exercise being preformed. The more anaerobic the exercise the better it is, ex. sprints. When exercise is maintained above the lactic acid threshold for more than 10 minutes, HGH will be released both during the exercise and periodically over the following 24 hours.[45]

Melatonin

Melatonin is a hormone secreted by the pineal gland in the brain.

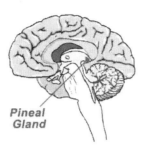

Pineal Gland

It helps regulate other hormones and maintains the body's circadian rhythm. The circadian rhythm is an internal 24-hour "clock" that plays a critical role in when we fall asleep and when we wake up. When it is dark, your body produces more melatonin; when it is light, the production of melatonin drops.

Being exposed to bright lights in the evening or too little light during the day can disrupt the body's normal melatonin cycles. For example, jet lag, shift work, and poor vision can disrupt melatonin cycles.

Some researchers also believe that melatonin levels may be related to aging. For example, young children have the highest levels of nighttime melatonin. Researchers believe these levels drop as we age. Some people think lower levels of melatonin may explain why some older adults have sleep problems and tend to go to bed and wake up earlier than when they were younger.[46]

Dr. William Regelson in his book The Super Hormone Promise "states that the groundbreaking work of Dr. Walter Pierpaoli has shown that the pineal gland is the body's aging clock."

By age 45, melatonin begins its steepest decline and the pineal gland begins to lose the cells necessary to produce melatonin.

By age 60 we produce half the amount of melatonin we produced at age twenty. "

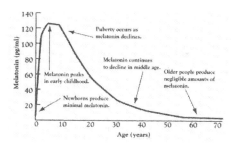

In a groundbreaking experiment, Dr. Pierpaoli removed the pineal glands from young mice and transplanted them into older mice and removed the pineal glands from the same older mice and transplanted them into the same younger mice, essentially switching the pineal glands between the older and younger mice.

The results were startling in that the older mice with young pineal glands were getting younger and the younger mice with the old pineal glands were rapidly aging, showing that the pineal gland may indeed be the bodies' aging clock. The same results were verified by experiments at Tel Aviv University and Hebrew University Hadassah Medical School and Spain's University of La Laguna!

Dr. Regelson states that "from this experiment Walter had his long sought proof that he had found the aging clock and had finally unlocked the mysterious mechanism that determines not only *how* we age, but *why* we age. By restoring melatonin to youthful levels, we are bringing the pineal gland back to its youthful state, and in doing so, we alter the message that it sends out to the rest of the body."

> Dr. Regelson goes on to state that "melatonin enhances the immune system and may possibly help restore the Thymus gland.
>
> The Thymus is a small gland located behind the breastbone where infection fighting T cells are stored.
>
> It also strengthens antibody response to fight off unwanted invaders, fights viruses, blocks the damage caused by stress, may possibly help treat some cancers, protect against heart disease and help you sleep!"[47]

Dr. Regelson and Dr. Pierpaoli recommend the following dosage for anti-aging.

AGE	Dose of Melatonin
40-45	.5 mg to 1 mg at bedtime
45-55	1 mg to 2 mg at bedtime
55-65	2 mg to 2.5 mg at bedtime
65-75	2.5 mg to 5 mg at bedtime
75 plus	3.5 mg to 5 mg at bedtime.[48]

Authors note: Dosing melatonin is a trial and error process. You should begin with ½ mg for several days and increase every few days by ½ mg until the desired sleep effect is reached. If you feel groggy the next day decrease the dosage by ½ mg.

Getting blood levels of Melatonin is a bit more difficult that other hormones due to the fact that Melatonin is secreted at night!

Melatonin is sold over the counter in various strengths.

Vitamins and Minerals

Any discussion of anti-aging must touch on the role vitamins and minerals play.

Why do we need vitamins and minerals?

As we keep stating, everything slows down with age. This is something we hate to admit, but cannot deny. The body slows down and becomes less efficient because cell generation slows down.

With all this slowing down, we also have to deal with nutritional deficiencies well in advance. As we age, we start eating less, which means less nutrition and vitamins and minerals go into our bodies.

On top of this, chronic diseases and medication can also affect the vitamin and mineral balance in the body. This is when we start feeling less than what we are. This is why we need vitamins and minerals. It is beneficial getting the required vitamins and minerals in supplementation form.[48]

It is also worth noting that the nutritional value of the foods we eat today does not contain the same value as it did in the past. Farming methods, processing, storage, and shipping diminish the amount of vitamins and minerals in our food.

Vitamins are organic molecules that the body needs to carry out its normal functions. Minerals are essential in building the body cells. The body needs vitamins and minerals in order to grow, repair tissue, fight off disease, and to stay healthy.

Each vitamin and mineral plays a specific role in the human body.

Everyday our body manufactures billions of red blood cells and approximately every 4 months our blood supply is totally renewed. About every 1-3 months our skin regenerates and about every 90 days our bones are rebuilt. In order to carry this out, an ample supply of vitamins and minerals are necessary.

Vitamins:

There are two types of vitamins: fat soluble and water soluble. Fat soluble vitamins are stored in the fat tissues and liver. The fat soluble vitamins include vitamin A, D, E and K.
Water soluble vitamins are not stored. Water soluble vitamins need to be replenished every day. These include the vitamin B group and vitamin C.

Minerals:

Minerals are as important as vitamins in the body and they have a multi-functional role. They are found in the entire body. There are two types of minerals - essential minerals and trace elements.

The essential minerals are calcium, iron, magnesium, sodium, potassium, phosphorous, and sulfur. The trace elements include boron, cobalt, copper, chromium, fluoride, iodine, manganese, molybdenum, selenium, silicon and zinc.

Minerals play an important role in activating enzymes in the body. A deficiency of any mineral may lead to acute or chronic ailments ex. a decrease in potassium and magnesium may lead to heart attacks. Minerals help prevent diseases such as osteoporosis, cancer, arthritis, anemia, goiter, periodontal disease and gastrointestinal problems.

Potassium, sodium, iron and calcium are essential in nerve formations and are needed for controlling fluids in and out of the cells. They are important in converting food into energy. If a single mineral is deficient, it will affect the proper functioning of the body. Minerals help control the way the body uses proteins, carbohydrates, fats and vitamins. Without minerals the body cannot work efficiently.

Following is a chart of the vitamins and minerals with information regarding each!

Vitamin/Mineral		What it does
Vitamin A (Retinol or Beta-carotene)		Keeps eyes healthy; develops bones; protects linings of respiratory, digestive and urinary tracts; maintains healthy skin and hair. Beta carotene fights free radicals (chemicals that damage cells).
Vitamin B_1 (Thiamine)		Promotes healthy functioning of the nerves, muscles and heart. Metabolizes carbohydrates.
Vitamin B_2 (Riboflavin)		Metabolizes carbohydrates, fats and proteins, produces hormones; promotes eye and skin health.
Vitamin B_3 (Niacin)		Metabolizes carbohydrates and fats; helps functioning of digestive system; maintains health skin.

Vitamin B$_5$ (Pantothenic Acid)		Produces hormones and maintains body's immune system.
Vitamin B$_6$ (Pyridoxine)		Metabolizes protein; helps produce hemoglobin; promotes functioning of digestive and nervous systems, and healthy skin.
Vitamin B$_{12}$ (Cyanocobalamin)		Builds genetic material of cells and produces blood cells.
Vitamin C (Ascorbic Acid)		An antioxidant, fights and resists infection; heals wounds; promotes growth and maintenance of bones, teeth, gums, ligaments and blood vessels.
Vitamin D (Cholecalciferol)		Builds strong bones and teeth and maintains the nervous system.
Vitamin E (Tocopherol)		Protects the lungs, nervous system, skeletal muscle and

		the eye's retina from damage by free radicals; may reduce risk of heart disease by protecting against atherosclerosis.
Vitamin H (Biotin)		Metabolizes proteins and carbohydrates; breaks down fatty acids.
Vitamin K		Promotes normal blood-clotting.
Vitamin M (Folic Acid)		Synthesis of protein and genetic materials; may help prevent some cancers, heart disease and stroke; when taken during pregnancy, protects against some birth defects.
Calcium (Ca)		Builds bones and teeth; promotes blood clotting, contraction of muscles and nerve impulses.
Chromium (Cr)		An essential nutrient required for normal

		sugar and fat metabolism; may also help prevent high cholesterol and atherosclerosis.
Copper (Cu)		Builds bones, red blood cells and hemoglobin; metabolizes iron, maintains connective tissue and blood vessels; may play a role in cancer prevention.
Fluoride (F)		Promotes bone and tooth formation; prevents tooth decay.
Iodine (I$_2$)		Helps produce thyroid hormones; adequate iodine intake during pregnancy is crucial to normal fetal development.
Iron (Fe)		Helps produce hemoglobin and red blood cells; delivers oxygen to muscles and other body tissues; protects against effects of

		stress
Magnesium (Mg)		Builds bones and teeth; involved in functioning of muscular and nervous systems and hear and circulatory system.
Manganese (Mn)		Involved in reproductive processes, sex hormone formation; essential for normal brain function and bone development.
Molybdenum (Mo)		Involved in enzyme activities.
Phosphorus (P)		Builds bones and teeth.
Potassium (K)		Helps nerves and muscles function; regulates heart's rhythm; regulates bodily fluids.
Selenium (Se)		An antioxidant, helps protect cells and tissues from damage by free radicals; may

			also protect against some cancers.

Along with all the above mentioned vitamins and minerals, which we need, there are certain ones that play a bigger role in the area of anti-aging. Some are listed below.

Resveratrol:

Resveratrol has been the subject of some of the most exciting anti-aging research. The health benefits of red wine can be attributed to this molecule.

Resveratrol anti-aging power lies in the fact that it can activate a class of longevity genes found in the body that are known as sirtuins.

Sirtuins reduce cellular damage while imparting greater power to your cells for repairing themselves. Many scientists suggest that this type of gene exists in all forms of living organisms and the benefits they bring can be likened to calorie restricted diets – enhance cellular respiration and boost your body's metabolism.

Resveratrol is also believed to be responsible for the so-called French Paradox – where the French possess far better heart health then would be expected from their diet and lifestyle.

Resveratrol well-researched free radical quenching abilities have been shown to support the health of a broad range of body tissues, organs and systems, including the cardiovascular and nervous systems.

Green Tea Extract:

EGCG (Epigallocatechin Gallate), one of the most powerful naturally occurring antioxidants, which has been scientifically linked to the traditional benefits of green tea, continues to be the subject of some of the most exciting anti-aging research relating to the heart, brain and other vital organs.

This should rank very high as an anti-aging supplement.

In addition to it being a very potent antioxidant, it also supports and enhances the activity of our body's own internal antioxidants, which are vital to our health. EGCG also supports a healthy immune system.

EGCG has been found to decrease the risk of developing atherosclerosis. It has strong anti-inflammatory properties and thereby decreases arterial inflammation which decreases the chances of sticky build up on the artery walls.

This could also lower blood pressure as it eases the heart's task of pumping blood through less inflamed arteries. We can slow the process of aging through the use of EGCG because of its ability to reduce, eliminate and neutralize free radicals and the damage they cause. EGCG may help you improve overall health because of its antioxidant abilities to strengthen, repair and optimize cellular health.

CoQ10:

There are numerous CoQ10 benefits. CoQ10 has long been accepted as necessary for all cellular energy production and must also be present in every cell in our body. All cells require it to produce energy and provide powerful antioxidant protection.

Overall, ninety-five percent of the human body's energy requirements are met with the energy converted in processes involving it. CoQ10 is sometimes also referred to as *ubiquinol*, a name formed with the word ubiquitous (which means "being or seeming to be everywhere at the same time; omnipresent"), because coenzyme Q10 is found in virtually every cell in the body.

CoQ10 is found in the highest concentrations in the hardest working organs in the body, such as the heart, brain, liver and kidneys.

The ability of these organs to produce energy and protect themselves from free radicals defines what good health and anti-aging supplements are all about.

Researchers have demonstrated that CoEnzyme Q10 deficiencies are more prevalent with age. As we grow older, we are no longer able to produce CoQ10 from the food in our diet.

As we age, the body loses its efficiency in manufacturing important nutrients. Therefore, even though the young may be able to get enough CoQ10 by making it and ingesting it through diet, a gradual deficiency may develop as we reach middle age and beyond. In addition, people with serious diseases (such as heart disease and cancer) tend to have low CoQ10 levels. Consumed regularly, Coenzyme Q10 fights off the aging process as it contributes to greater health and longevity. [50]

Many physicians are warning that Statin drugs can lower levels of CoQ10.

Dr. Mercola states, "Ironically, while reducing your risk of cardiovascular events and heart disease is the primary motivation for prescribing statins, these drugs can actually increase your risk of heart disease.

They deplete your body of Coenzyme Q10 (CoQ10), which can lead to heart failure. **Statins lower your CoQ10 levels by blocking the pathway involved in cholesterol production – the same pathway by which Q10 is produced.**"[51]

Omega 3:

The Omega-3 oils make up billions and billions of cell membranes in our body and since they cannot be made by the body, their health benefits are only available by eating a diet rich in fish or with an Omega-3 supplement.

Its importance in heart, brain and circulatory health make it a dynamic anti-aging supplement.

They help lower cholesterol, triglycerides, LDLs and blood pressure, while at the same time increasing good HDL cholesterol. This adds years to your life expectancy.

Research has shown that diets rich in Omega-3 fats are associated with superior heart, brain and circulator health. Unfortunately, the typical American diet supplies little of the Omega-3's necessary or suggested for good health. The Omega-3 benefits come from DHA (Docosahexaenoic Acid) and EPA (Eicosapentaenoic Acid). In addition to the heart benefits of DHA and EPA, DHA has been shown to be very important in brain and eye function. Both EPA and DHA are vital to the structure and function of the brain, but the highest function areas of the brain contain very high levels of DHA.

Alpha Lipoic Acid:

Alpha Lipoic Acid has the rare ability to exist in either water or oil-based environments. This enables ALA to deliver its powerful antioxidant benefits anywhere in the body. It is this universal solubility that results in ALA being commonly referred to as the "universal antioxidant".

ALA's solubility allows it to be particularly effective in providing its antioxidant benefits to the cells of our nervous system and brain where its chemical structure allows it to cross the blood-brain-barrier.

About forty years ago, biologists discovered that ALA is also an antioxidant, a powerful substance that combats potentially harmful chemicals called free radicals, which may cause heart and liver disease, cancer, cell aging and many other conditions.

There are other very effective antioxidants, including vitamins C and E. Scientists believe that ALA operates in conjunction with vitamins C and E and the antioxidant glutathione, recycling them when they're used up. Many studies have been conducted confirming the health benefits of alpha lipoic acid, including recent findings that ALA offers neuroprotective and possibly cognitive enhancing effects. Unfortunately, the body makes very low concentrations of ALA and like many of the vital substances that we rely upon our bodies to produce; we may need to consume more Alpha Lipoic Acid supplements due to the normal changes accompanying aging, stress, illness and even exercise.

Gama Tocopherol:

Major form of Vitamin E found in nature – Millions of people consume Vitamin E supplements for its powerful antioxidant benefits and gamma tocopherol is the most potent antioxidant among all four forms of this vitamin.

Since alpha tocopherol has historically been the major type of Vitamin E manufactured and sold, gamma tocopherol received very little attention.

The combination of Vitamin E alpha and gamma tocopherol is a much more potent antioxidant than alpha-tocopherol alone.

Gamma tocopherol has also been shown to support the activity of alpha tocopherol, as well as other benefits of its own. Gamma Vitamin E supplementation can result in an increase in alpha tocopherol concentrations in the body, whereas taking alpha only may lessen or suppress gamma tocopherol. These two forms work together nicely to create a strong antioxidant benefit. All four forms of Vitamin E can be found in our diet, but only in foods that we consume very little of such as high fat, high calorie vegetable oils, margarines and shortenings. As a result, the Vitamin E content in our diet is extremely low. Also, as noted above, most Vitamin E supplements only deliver alpha tocopherol, which is less beneficial than gamma tocopherol.

Most vitamin E benefits are experiences with the Gamma form. Research continues on the role of Gamma Vitamin E in the reduction of breast cancer, prostate cancer and colon cancer. Gamma Vitamin E is a potent destroyer of free radicals in the body, therefore making it a great anti-aging supplement to consume.[50]

Summary

As stated previously, entire books can and have been written on each hormone and on the vitamins and minerals.

We hope you will take the information we have presented, find an anti-aging physician and get all your required blood tests taken to make sure you have adequate levels of all the male hormones, vitamins and minerals or at least research more into areas that, you feel, may benefit you. We are providing you with some resources that may help you in this endeavor.

As always consult with an anti-aging physician before initiating any hormone therapy or vitamin, mineral supplementation.

RESOURCES

Resource Books:

- The Thyroid Solution, Ridha Arem M.D.

- The Complete Thyroid Book, Kenneth Ain M.D., Sarah Rosenthal, Ph D

- Hypothyroidism, Type 2, Mark Starr M.D.

- Hypothyroidism, The Unsuspected Illness, Broda Barnes, M.D.

- The DHEA Breakthrough, Stephen Cherniske, M.S.

- The Metabolic Plan, Stephen Cherniske, M.S.

- DHEA, a Practical Guide, Ray Sahelian, M.D.

- Stopping the Clock, Ronald Klatz, M.D., Robert Goldman, M.D.

- The Miracle of Natural Hormones, David Brownstein, M.D.

- The Testosterone Syndrome, Eugene Shippen, M.D.

- Testosterone for Life, Abraham Morgenthaler, M.D.

- The Life Extension Revolution, Phillip Lee Miller, M.D.

- The Super Hormone Promise, William Regelson, M.D.

- The Melatonin Miracle, Walter Pierpaoli, M.D. & William Regelson, M.D.

Anti-Aging Resource

Local Physician

Dr. Jeffery Brown,

10120 S. Eastern Ave. Henderson, NV

optimalhealthpc.com

The American Academy of Anti-Aging Medicine www.a4m.com

Homeopathic HGH Spray

www.21stcenturyhgh.com

fountainofyout@aol.com

REFERENCES

1 medical-dictionary.thefreedictionary.com/aging

2 www.future-of-anti-aging.com/anti-aging-research.html

3 Steadman's Medical Dictionary

4 Hanukoglu I (Dec 1992). "Steroidogenic enzymes: structure, function, and role in regulation of steroid hormone biosynthesis.". *J Steroid Biochem Mol Biol* 43 (8): 779–804. doi:10.1016/0960-0760(92)90307-5. PMID 22217824\

5 "National Health and Nutrition Examination Survey" (PDF). United States Center for Disease Control. Retrieved 2012-01-28.

6 Lecerf JM, de Lorgeril M (2011). "Dietary cholesterol: from physiology to cardiovascular risk". *Br J Nutr* 106 (1): 6–14. doi:10.1017/S0007114511000237. PMID 21385506

7 renewman.com/male-hormones/why-hormones-decline

8 answers.yahoo.com/question/index?qid

=20090111210728AAcWxP6

9 medicinenet.com/hypothyroidism/article.htm Thyroid gland pic

10 medterms.com/script/main/

art.asp?articlekey=577

11 andlos.com/thyroid-disease "The American Association of Clinical Endocrinologists "

12 Level of thyroid hormone chart

13 Pathway chart mdlongevity.com/pro-h-thyroid.html

14 mdlongevity.com/pro-h-thyroid.html

15 allonhealth.com/hypothyroidism-test.htm

16 Hypothyroidism Type 2: The Epidemic.

17 www.21centurymed.com

18 Hypothyroidism : The Unsuspected Illness Broda O. Barnes

19 en.wikipedia.org/wiki/

DehyDroepianDrosterone

20 livestrong.com/article/474382-dhea-vs-dhea-s

21 nlm.nih.gov/medlineplus/ency/

article/003717.htm

22 www.vanderbilt.edu/AnS/

psychology/health_psychology/DHEA

23 www.lefeurope.com/en/concerns/dhea-restoration-therapy

24 www.anti-agingmd.com/dhea.html

25 www.dheausa.com/immune_system.htm

26 www.prweb.com/releases/2013/3/ prweb10508748.htm

27 www.lefeurope.com/en/concerns/dhea-restoration-therapy

28 Testosterone for Life, Abraham Morgentaler, M.D.

29 www.everydayhealth.com/mens-health/...low-testosterone.aspx

30 nationwidesi.com/for_men.cfm

31 prohormonedb.com/content.asp?t=

What+is%3A+Aromatase

32 www.lef.org/magazine/...Know-Your-Sex-Hormone-Status_01.htm

33 www.lowtestosteronetreatmentsite.com/low-testosterone

34 http://www.med-health.net/Herbs-For-Testosterone.html

35 http://www.newhealthguide.org/High-Estrogen-In-Men.html

36 http://www.quickanddirtytips.com/health-fitness/mens-health/6-ways-to-increase-testosterone-with-exercise

37 en.wikipedia.org/wiki/Growth_hormone

38 www.hghmeds.org/the-history-of-hgh

39www.discountghr15.com/info/rudman-hgh-study.php

40 www.webmd.com/balance/guide/

homeopathy-topic-overview

41 www.homeopathic-hgh.com

42 Feeling Younger with Homeopathic HGH

43 Howard Davis: Feeling Younger with Homeopathic HGH

44 http://www..com/articles/naturally-boost- muscleand strength growth-hormone- testosterone

45 www.livestrong.com/.../191932-ways-to-boost-growth-hormones

46 http://www.webmd.com/sleep-disorders/tc/melatonin-overview

47 "The Super Hormone Promise", Dr William Regelson

48 irefuse2age.com

49 The American Society for Nutritional Sciences Nutrient Information

50 anti-aging-supplement-guide.com

51 mercola.com

52 www.isitlowt.com/do-you-have-low-t/low-t-quiz

Made in the USA
Lexington, KY
16 February 2014